Best Low-Carb Recipes for your Ketogenic Bread

50 super delicious recipes for your ketogenic bread to stay healthy and boost energy

Raul Wyatt

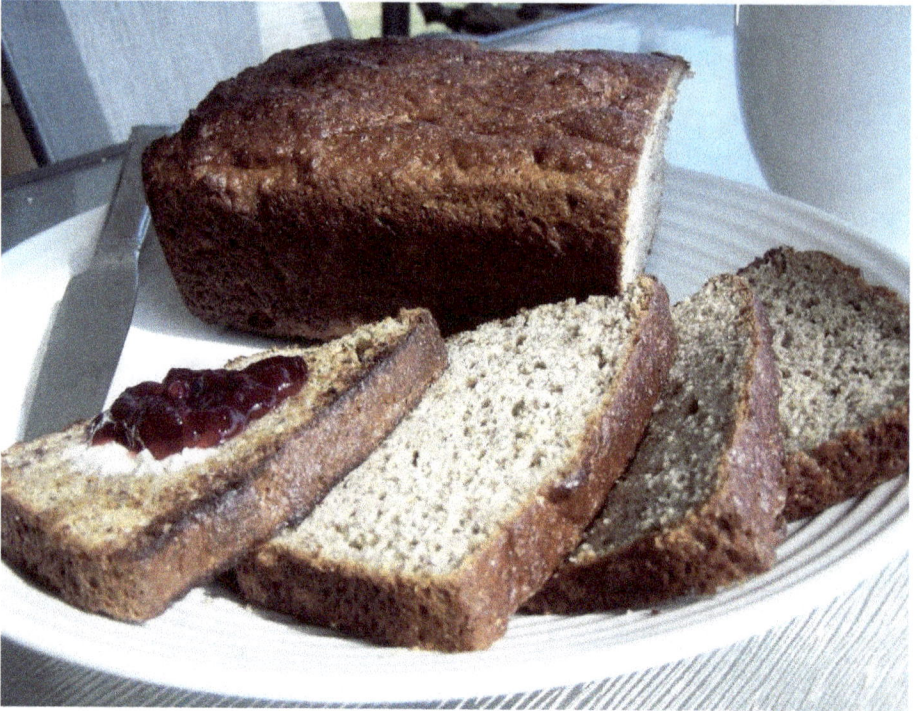

COPYRIGHT

Table of Contents

German Black Bread

Preparation time: 3 hours

Cooking time: 50 minutes

Servings: 10

Ingredients:

· 1 cup water plus 2 tablespoons water

· 2 tablespoons apple cider vinegar

· 2 tablespoons molasses

· 1 tablespoon sugar

· 1 teaspoon salt

· 1 teaspoon instant coffee

· ¼ teaspoon fennel seeds

· 1 tablespoon caraway seeds

· ½ ounce unsweetened chocolate

· ½ cup bran cereal flakes

· ½ cup bread flour

· ½ cup rye flour

· 2 cups whole almond flour

· 1 package active dry yeast

Directions:

1. Put all of the bread ingredients in your bread machine in the order listed above starting with the water, and finishing with the yeast. Set the bread machine to the Whole wheat function.

2. Check on the dough after about 5 minutes and make sure that it's a soft ball. Add water 1 tablespoon at a time if it's too dry, and add flour 1 tablespoon at a time if it's too wet.

3. When the bread is done allow it to cool on a wire rack.

Nutrition:

· Calories: 102

· Carbohydrates: 3.8 g

· Fiber: 3.4 g

· Fat:: 1.4 g

· Protein: 5.0 g

Hazelnut Honey Bread

Preparation time: 3 hours

Cooking time: 30 minutes

Servings: 10

Ingredients:

· ½ cup lukewarm milk

· 2 teaspoons butter, melted and cooled

· 2 teaspoons liquid honey

· 2/3 teaspoon salt

· 1/3 cup cooked wild rice, cooled

· 1/3 cup whole grain flour

· 2/3 teaspoons caraway seeds

· 1 cup almond flour, sifted

· 1 teaspoon active dry yeast

· 1/3 cup hazelnuts, chopped

Directions:

1. Prepare all of the ingredients for your bread and measuring utensils (a cup, a spoon, kitchen scales).

2. Carefully measure the ingredients into the pan, except the nuts and seeds.

3. Place all of the ingredients into the bread bucket in the right order, following the manual for your bread machine.

4. Close the cover.

5. Select the program of your bread machine to Basic and choose the crust color to Medium.

6. Press Start.

7. After the signal, add the nuts and seeds into the dough.

8. Wait until the program completes.

9. When done, take the bucket out and let it cool for 5-10 minutes.

10. Shake the loaf from the pan and let it cool for 30 minutes on a cooling rack.

11. Slice, serve, and enjoy the taste of fragrant homemade bread.

Nutrition:

· Carbohydrates: 5 g

· Fats: 2.8 g

· Protein: 3.6 g

· Calories: 113

Pita Bread

Preparation time: 10 minutes

Cooking time: 15 minutes

Servings: 8

Ingredients:

• 2 cups almond flour, sifted

• ½ cup water

• 2 tablespoon olive oil

• Salt, to taste

• 1 teaspoon black cumin

Directions:

1. Preheat the oven to 400°F.

2. Combine the flour with salt. Add the water and olive oil.

3. Knead the dough and let it stand for 15 minutes.

4. Shape the dough into 8 balls.

5. Line a baking sheet with parchment paper and flatten the balls into 8 thin rounds.

6. Sprinkle black cumin.

7. Bake for 15 minutes, serve.

Nutrition:

· Calories: 73

· Fat: 6.9 g

· Carbohydrates: 1.6 g

· Protein: 1.6 g

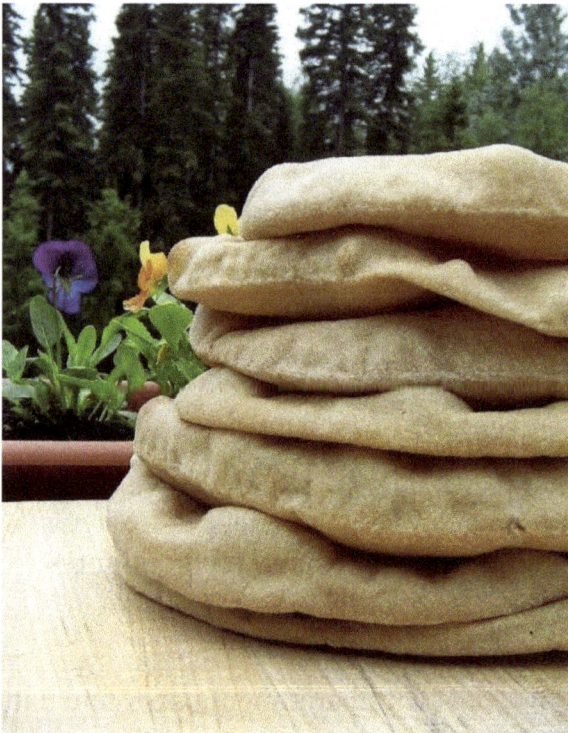

Pumpernickel Quick Bread

Preparation time: 30 minutes

Cooking time: 35 minutes

Servings: 1 loaf

Ingredients:

· 1/2 cup cassava flour or whole wheat flour

· 1/2 cup water

· 1 1/2 cups almond flour

· 4 eggs

· 1 1/2 tablespoons cacao/cocoa powder

· 2 tablespoons molasses

· 1 tablespoon baking powder

· 2 tablespoons butter, melted

· 1 tablespoon brown sugar

· 1 teaspoon salt

· 2 tablespoons caraway seeds

Directions:

1.Add all ingredients to the Bread Machine.

2.Smooth out the top of the loaf. Choose Quick Bread mode and press Start. Let it bake for about 35 minutes.

3.Remove bread from the bread machine and let it rest for 10 minutes. Enjoy!

Nutrition:

· Calories:192

· Fat: 5.6 g

· Total carbohydrates: 33 g

· Protein: 4 g

Paleo Coconut Bread

Preparation time: 10 minutes

Cooking time: 50 minutes

Servings: 10

Ingredients:

· ½ cup coconut flour

· ¼ cup almond milk (unsweetened)

· ¼ cup coconut oil (melted)

· 6 eggs

· ¼ teaspoon baking soda

· ¼ teaspoon salt

Directions:

1.Preheat the oven to 350°F.

2.Line an (8 x 4) loaf pan with parchment paper.

3.In a bowl, combine salt, baking soda, and coconut flour.

4.Combine the oil, milk, and eggs in another bowl.

5.Gradually add the wet ingredients into the dry ingredients and mix well.

6.Pour the mixture into the prepared loaf pan.

7.Bake for 40 to 50 minutes.

8.Cool, slice, and serve.

Nutrition:

· Calories: 108

· Fat: 8.7 g

· Carbohydrates: 3.4 g

· Protein: 4.2 g

Collagen Bread

Preparation time: 30 minutes

Cooking time: 3 hours

Servings: 12

Ingredients:

· 6 tablespoons almond flour

· ½ cup collagen protein, unflavored

· 1 teaspoon baking powder

· 1 teaspoon Xanthan gum

· pinch of pink salt

· 5 eggs, separated

· 1 tablespoon coconut oil, unflavored and liquid

Directions:

1. Add all the ingredients to the Bread machine.

2. Close the lid and choose Bread mode. Once done, take out from the machine and cut into at least 16 slices.

Nutrition:

· Calories:77

Fluffy Buns

Preparation time: 1 hour

Cooking time: 30 minutes

Servings: 4

Ingredients:

· ¼ cup almond flour

· 1 tablespoon psyllium husk powder

· ¼ cup coconut flour

· sesame seeds

· 1 teaspoon baking powder

· 1 egg

· 3 egg whites

· ¼ cup boiling hot water

Directions:

1. Add all ingredients to the Bread Machine.

2. Select Dough setting. When the time is over, transfer the dough to the floured surface. Shape it into a ball. Separate dough into 4 portions and make buns.

3. Line a baking sheet with parchment paper, place on it, and add sesame seeds on top. Make a cut on the top.

4. Heat the oven to 356°F and bake for 25 minutes.

Nutrition:

· Calories: 109

· Fat: 5.5 g

· Total carbohydrates: 8.3 g

· Protein: 7.3 g

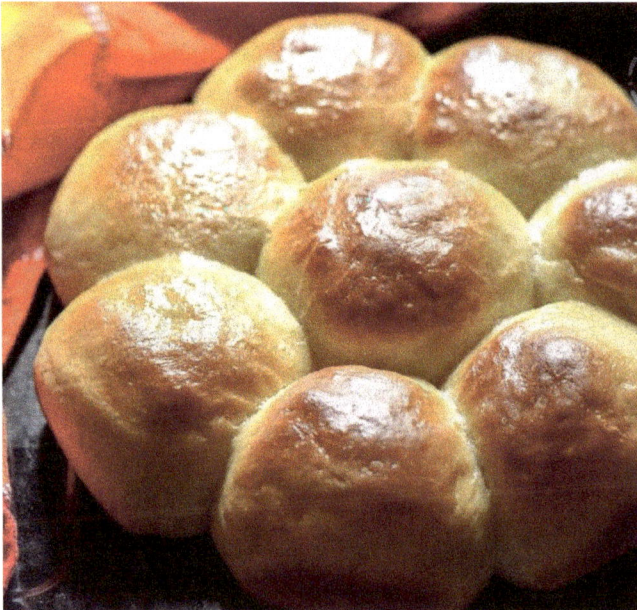

Yeasted Avocado Bread

Preparation time: 3 hours

Cooking time: 22 minutes

Servings: 10

Ingredients:

· 2 ½ teaspoons active dry yeast

· 1 teaspoon Erythritol

· 2 teaspoons baking powder

· 1/3 cup golden flax meal

· ½ cup almond flour

· ¼ cup whole psyllium husk

· 1 teaspoon sea salt

· ½ cup hot water

· 4 eggs

· 1 avocado

· ¼ cup extra water

· 2 tablespoons olive oil

Directions:

1. Add water, yeast, and Erythritol to the bread machine and let rest there for 10 minutes.

2. Add the remaining ingredients and select Bread mode on the machine.

3. After the cooking time is over, remove the bread from the machine and let it rest for about 10 minutes. Enjoy!

Nutrition:

· Calories: 101

· Fat: 8.3 g

· Total carbohydrates: 3 g

· Protein: 4 g

Keto Kalamata Olive Loaf

Preparation time: 2 hours

Cooking time: 10 minutes

Total Time: 2 hours 10 minutes

Servings: 10 slices

Ingredients:

· ½ cup brine from olives

· 1 cup warm water

· 2 tablespoons olive oil

· 1 ½ teaspoon salt

· 2 tablespoons sugar

· 3 cups almond flour

· 1 2/3 cup almond meal

· 1 ½ teaspoons dried basil leaves

· 2 teaspoons active dry yeast

· ½ cup olives finely chopped

Directions:

1.Combine the brine and warm water.

2.Using the bread bucket, put all ingredients except olives in the order of their appearance on the ingredient list, starting with the brine mixture.

3.Select the Wheat Bread cycle on your machine. If there is no Wheat Bread cycle, you can select the Basic cycle. Close the cover and press Start.

4.With the first beep of the machine, open the lid and add in the olives. Close the lid and let the cycle continue.

5.When the cycle ends, you can take the loaf out and let it cool in a cooling rack.

6.Slice before serving.

Nutrition:

· Calories: 161

· Calories from fat: 130

· Total Fat: 14 g

· Total Carbohydrates: 8 g

· Net Carbohydrates: 5 g

· Protein: 5 g

Rosemary and Garlic Bread

Preparation time: 10 minutes

Cooking time: 50 minutes

Servings: 8

Ingredients:

· 1/2 cup coconut flour

· 1 stick butter (8 tablespoon)

· 6 large eggs

· 1 teaspoon baking powder

· 2 teaspoons dried rosemary

· 1/2-1 teaspoon garlic powder

· 1/2 teaspoon onion powder

· 1/4 teaspoon pink Himalayan salt

Direction:

1.Start by whisking rosemary, salt, garlic, onion, baking powder, and coconut flour in a bowl.

2.Beat eggs in a mixing bowl until creamy.

3.Now, put butter in a large bowl and melt it in the microwave.

4.Slowly stir in the whisked eggs and continue beating with a hand mixer.

5.Now, whisk in the dry mixture and mix well until well incorporated.

6.Spread the batter in an 8x4 inch loaf pan and bake it for 50 minutes approximately at 350 °F.

7.Slice and serve with butter on top.

Nutrition:

· Calories: 214

· Total Fat: 19 g

· Saturated Fat: 5.8 g

· Total Carbohydrates: 6.5 g

· Sugar: 1.9 g

· Fiber: 2.1 g

· Protein: 6.5 g

Parsley Cheddar Bread

Preparation time: 10 minutes

Cooking time: 4 minutes

Servings: 2

Ingredients:

· 1 tablespoon butter

· 2 tablespoons coconut flour

· 1 large egg

· 1 tablespoon heavy whipping cream

· 2 tablespoons water

· 1/4 cup Cheddar cheese

· 1/8 teaspoon garlic powder

· 1/8 teaspoon onion powder

· 1/8 teaspoon dried parsley

· 1/8 teaspoon pink Himalayan salt

· 1/8 teaspoon black pepper

· 1/4 teaspoon baking powder

Direction:

1.Melt the butter by heating it in a coffee mug for 20 seconds.

2.Slowly stir in seasonings, baking powder, and coconut flour. Mix well using a fork until smooth.

3.Whisk in cream, cheese, water, and egg.

4.Beat well until smooth, then bake for 3 minutes in the microwave.

5.Allow the bread to cool, then serve.

Nutrition:

· Calories: 113

· Total Fat: 8.4 g

· Saturated Fat: 12.1 g

· Total Carbohydrates: 9.2 g

· Sugar. 3.1 g

· Fiber: 4.6 g

· Protein. 8.1 g

Almond Bread

Preparation time: 10 minutes

Cooking time: 30 minutes

Servings: 10

Ingredients:

· 1 1/2 cups almond flour

· 6 large eggs, separated

· 1/4 cup butter, melted

· 3 teaspoons baking powder

· 1/4 teaspoon cream of tartar

· 1 pinch pink Himalayan salt

· 6 drops liquid stevia

Directions:

1. Start by preheating your oven to 375 °F.

2. Now, separate the egg yolks from their whites.

3. Beat the whites with cream of tartar in a mixing bowl until it's foamy and creamy.

4.Blend egg yolks with butter, almond flour, salt, baking powder, stevia, and 1/3 of the egg white mixture in a food processor.

5.Once blended well, fold in the remaining egg whites, then transfer the batter to a greased 8x4 loaf pan.

6.Bake the bread for 30 minutes or until it's done.

7.Slice into 20 slices and serve fresh.

Nutrition:

· Calories: 107

· Total Fat: 9.3 g

· Saturated Fat:.4.8 g

· Total Carbohydrates: 2.6 g

· Fiber: 0.8 g

· Protein: 3.9 g

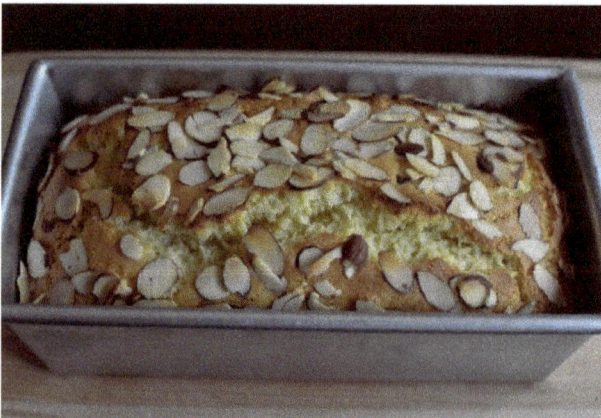

Psyllium Husk Bread

Preparation time: 10 minutes

Cooking time: 35 minutes

Servings: 10

Ingredients:

· 1/2 cup coconut flour

· 2 tablespoons psyllium husk powder

· 1/2 teaspoon baking powder

· 1/4 teaspoon pink Himalayan salt

· 3/4 cup water

· 4 large eggs

· 4 tablespoons butter

Direction:

1.Start by whisking the husk powder, salt, baking powder, and coconut flour in a bowl.

2.Beat eggs with water and melted butter in a mixer until it is smooth.

3.Slowly stir in the dry mixture and mix well until smooth.

4.Make 10 dinner rolls out of this bread dough and place the dough on a baking sheet.

5.Bake them for 35 minutes, approximately, at 350 °F until all done.

6.Slice and serve.

Nutrition:

· Calories: 220

· Total Fat. 20.1 g

· Saturated Fat: 7.4 g

· Total Carbohydrates: 63 g

· Fiber: 2.4 g

· Protein: 6.1 g

Coconut Cloud Bread

Preparation time: 10 minutes

Cooking time: 25 minutes

Servings: 4

Ingredients:

· 3 eggs

· 3 tablespoons coconut cream

· 1/2 teaspoon baking powder

Optional toppings:

· Sea salt

· black pepper

· rosemary

Direction:

1.First, separate the egg yolks and egg whites.

2.Beat egg yolks in a bowl.

3.Stir in cream and continue beating with a hand mixer until creamy and smooth.

4.Beat the egg whites with baking powder in another bowl until it forms peaks.

5.Quickly add the yolk mixture to the whites and mix well until fluffy.

6.Spread ¼ of the batter onto a baking sheet separately to make 4 circles.

7.Bake the batter for 25 minutes approximately at 350 °F.

8.Serve.

Nutrition:

· Calories: 158

· Total Fat: 15.2 g

· Saturated Fat: 5.2 g

· Total Carbohydrates: 7.4 g

· Fiber: 3.5 g

· Protein: 5.5 g

Cloud Bread Loaf

Preparation time: 10 minutes

Cooking time: 15 minutes

Servings: 10

Ingredients:

· 6 egg whites

· 6 egg yolks

· 1/2 cup whey p rotein powder, unflavored

· 1/2 teaspoon cream of tartar

· 6 oz sour cream

· 1/2 teaspoon baking powder

· 1/4 teaspoon garlic powder

· 1/4 teaspoon onion powder

· 1/4 teaspoon salt

Directions:

1. Using a hand mixer, beat egg whites and cream of tartar together until you have stiff peaks forming. Set aside.

2. Combine all other ingredients into another bowl and mix together.

3. Fold the mixtures together, a little at a time.

4. Pour mixture into your bread machine pan.

5. Set the bread machine to Quick bread.

6. When the bread is done, remove the bread machine pan from the bread machine.

7. Let it cool slightly before transferring to a cooling rack.

8. The bread can be stored for up to 3 days on the counter.

Nutrition:

· Calories: 90

· Carbohydrates: 2 g

· Protein: 6 g

· Fat: 7 g

Almond Flour Bread

Preparation time: 10 minutes

Cooking time: 10 minutes

Servings: 10

Ingredients:

· 4 e gg whites

· 2 egg yolks

· 2 cups almond flour

· 1/4 cup butter, melted

· 2 tablespoons psyllium husk powder

· 1 1/2 teaspoon baking powder

· 1/2 teaspoon xanthan gum

· Salt

· 1/2 cup + 2 tablespoons w arm water

· 2 1/4 teaspoons yeast

Directions:

1. Use a small mixing bowl to combine all of the dry ingredients, except for the yeast.

2. In the bread machine pan, add all the wet ingredients .

3. Add all dry ingredients from the small mixing bowl into the bread machine pan. Top with the yeast.

4. Set the bread machine to the Basic bread setting.

5. When the bread is done, remove the bread machine pan from the bread machine.

6. Let it cool slightly before transferring to a cooling rack.

7. The bread can be stored for up to 4 days on the counter and for up to 3 months in the freezer.

Nutrition:

· Calories: 110

· Carbohydrates: 2.4 g

· Protein: 4 g

· Fat: 10 g

Pumpkin Bread for keto diet

Preparation time: 6 minutes

Cooking time: 21 min

Servings : 10

Ingredients:

· 1/2 cup spread, relaxed

· 2/3 cup erythritol sugar, similar to Swerve

· 4 eggs, large

· 3/4 cup pumpkin puree, canned (see notes for new)

· 1 teaspoon vanilla concentrate

· 1 1/2 cups almond flour

· 1/2 cup coconut flour

· 4 teaspoons preparing powder

· 1 teaspoon cinnamon

· 1/2 teaspoon nutmeg

· 1/4 teaspoon ginger

· 1/8 teaspoon cloves

· 1/2 teaspoon salt

Directions:

1. Preheat the stove to 350°F. Oil a 9"x5" portion skillet, and line with material paper.

2. In a big blending bowl, cream the margarine and sugar together until light and soft.

3. Add the eggs, each in turn, and blend well to consolidate.

4. Add the pumpkin puree and vanilla, and blend well to combine.

5. In a different bowl, mix together the almond flour, coconut flour, preparing powder, cinnamon, nutmeg, ginger, cloves, and salt. Separate any pieces of almond flour or coconut flour.

6. Add the dry ingredients to the wet ingredients, and mix to combine. (Alternatively, indicate 1/2 cup of blend ins, as cleaved nuts or chocolate chips.)

7. Pour the hitter into the readied portion dish. Prepare for 45–55 minutes, or until a toothpick inserted into the center of the portion comes out clean.

8. If the bread is sautéing too rapidly, you can cover the skillet with a bit of aluminum foil.

Nutrition:

· Calories: 50

· Carbohydrates: 12 g

· Net Carbs: 2.5 g

· Fiber: 4.5 g

Buttery Flatbread

Preparation time: 10 minutes

Cooking time: 8 minutes

Servings: 4

Ingredients:

· 1 cup almond flour

· 2 tablespoons coconut flour

· 2 teaspoons xanthan gum

· 1/2 teaspoon baking powder

· 1/2 teaspoon flaky salt

· 1 whole egg + 1 egg white

· 1 tablespoon water

· 1 tablespoon oil, for frying

· 1 tablespoon melted butter, for slathering

Direction:

1.Start by whisking baking powder, salt, flours, and xanthan gum in a bowl.

2.Beat egg whites and egg in a bowl until creamy.

3.Fold in flour mixture and mix until well incorporated.

4.Add a tablespoon of water to the dough and cut it into 4 equal parts.

5.Spread each part out into a flatbread and cook each for 1 minute per side in a skillet with oil.

6.Garnish with butter, parsley, and salt.

7.Serve.

Nutrition:

· Calories: 216

· Total Fat: 20.9 g

· Saturated Fat: 8.1 g

· Total Carbohydrates: 8.3 g

· Fiber: 3.8 g

· Protein: 6.4 g

Sweet Challah Bread for keto diet

Preparation time: 20 minutes

Cooking time: 3 hours

Total Time: 3 hours 20 minutes

Servings: 20 slices

Ingredients:

· 4 eggs

· 1 ½ ounces sukrin plus

· 12 ounces cream cheese

· 2 ounces butter

· 2 ounces heavy cream

· 1 ¾ ounces g vegetable oil

· 3 ½ ounces unflavored whey protein

· 3 ounces protein whey vanilla

· ½ teaspoon salt

· 3 g baking soda

· 12 g. baking powder

· 4 g xanthan

· ½ small lemon zest

· 1 ounce dried cranberries

Directions:

1.Place all ingredients on the bread machine pan except for lemon zest and cranberries.

2.Select the Sweet Bread cycle (or White Bread cycle) on the bread machine setting and Light on the Crust Color setting. Close the lid and press Start.

3.Just before the final rise, pause the bread machine and transfer the dough to a floured surface. Spread the dough and hand press the cranberries and lemon zest.

4.Divide the dough into three equal parts. Roll each part of the dough to a 10-inch long rope. Lay all three ropes parallel to each other and braid together gently. Tuck the ends to form an oblong loaf. Brush the dough with egg white.

5.Remove the kneading paddle of the bread machine before placing the dough back in the pan. Press the Start button again to resume the cycle.

6.Once the cycle is finished, you can remove the challah and transfer it to a cooling rack.

7.Slice and serve.

Nutrition:

· Calories: 158

· Calories from fat: 117

Coconut Flour Bread

Preparation time: 10 minutes

Cooking time: 15 minutes

Servings: 12

Ingredients:

· 6 eggs

· 1/2 cup coconut flour

· 2 tablespoons psyllium husk

· 1/4 cup olive oil

· 1 1/2 teaspoons salt

· 1 teaspoon xanthan gum

· 1 teaspoon baking powder

· 2 1/4 teaspoons yeast

Directions:

1. Use a small mixing bowl to combine all of the dry ingredients, except for the yeast.

2. In the bread machine pan, add all wet ingredients .

3. Add all dry ingredients, from the small mixing bowl to the bread machine pan. Top with the yeast.

4. Set the bread machine to the Basic bread setting.

5. When the bread is done, remove the bread machine pan from the bread machine.

6. Let it cool slightly before transferring to a cooling rack.

7. The bread can be stored for up to 4 days on the counter and for up to 3 months in the freezer.

Nutrition:

· Calories: 174

· Carbohydrates: 4 g

· Protein: 7 g

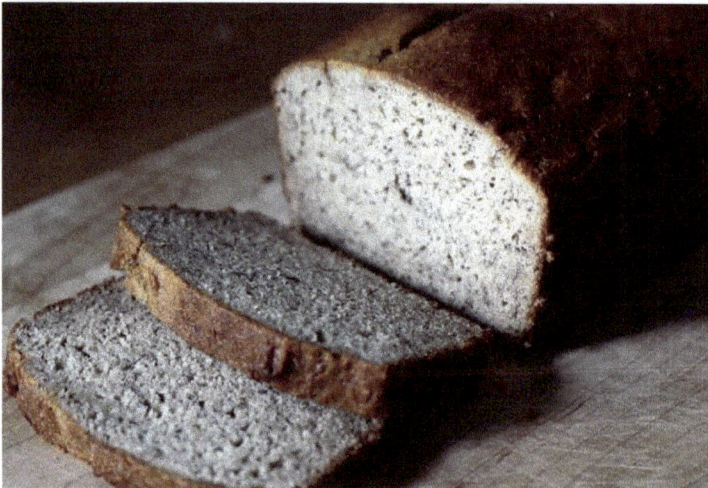

Keto Breakfast Meat Lovers Pizza

Preparation time: 90 minutes

Cooking time: 30 minutes

Total Time: 2 hours

Servings: 8 slices

Ingredients:

Crust

· 2 cups mozzarella cheese, shredded

· 2 tablespoons Cream cheese

· 1 egg

· ¾ cup almond flour

Toppings

· 6 eggs

· 2 tablespoons Heavy cream

· 1 tablespoon butter

· ½ cup crumbled bacon

· ½ cup cooked crumbled breakfast sausage

· ½ cup cheese sauce

· ¼ cup cheddar, shredded

· 2 tablespoons Green onions, chopped

Cheese Sauce

· 1 ¼ cup heavy whipping cream

· 2 oz. cream cheese

· 2 tablespoons Butter

· ½ teaspoon ground mustard

· ½ teaspoon pepper

· 6 oz. grated cheddar

· 3 oz. grated gruyere

Directions:

1.To start the crust, combine and melt the mozzarella and cream cheese in the microwave for 30 seconds.

2.Pour the cheese melted into the bread bucket, then add the eggs and almond flour. Place the bread bucket inside the bread machine.

3.Turn the bread machine on by selecting the Dough cycle, close the lid, then press start and wait for the cycle to finish in about 90 minutes.

4.While waiting for the dough, prepare the cheese sauce by combining whip cream, cream cheese, and butter in a saucepan over medium heat until melted.

5.Whisk in the mustard and pepper.

6.Remove from heat and whisk in the cheddar and gruyere until it turns creamy.

7.Preheat your oven at 425 °F before you start shaping the dough. Prepare a pizza pan and spray with non-stick baking spray. Set aside.

8.Roll your dough into a 12-inch diameter circle between 2 sheets of parchment paper.

9.Bake for 10 minutes until golden brown.

10. To do the sauce and toppings, whisk six eggs and cream in a bowl until combined.

11. Heat butter over medium fire in a large skillet. Add the egg mixture and scramble the egg until it turns a soft fluffy and slightly wet appearance.

12. Spread ½ cup of the cheese sauce onto the pizza crust, then topped with the scrambled egg, bacon, and sausage. Sprinkle the grated cheddar on top.

13. Return to the oven for another 5 minutes.

14. Remove from the oven and sprinkle green onions on top.

15. Slice and serve.

Notes:

16. The cheese sauce recipe yields 2 ½ cups and you only need ½ cup for the pizza. You can store the remaining sauce in an air-tight-lidded jar.

17. Recipe nutrition info includes the ½-cup cheese sauce.

Nutrition:

· Calories: 470

· Calories from fat: 333

· Total Fat: 37 g

· Total Carbohydrates: 4 g

· Net Carbohydrates: 3 g

· Protein: 28 g

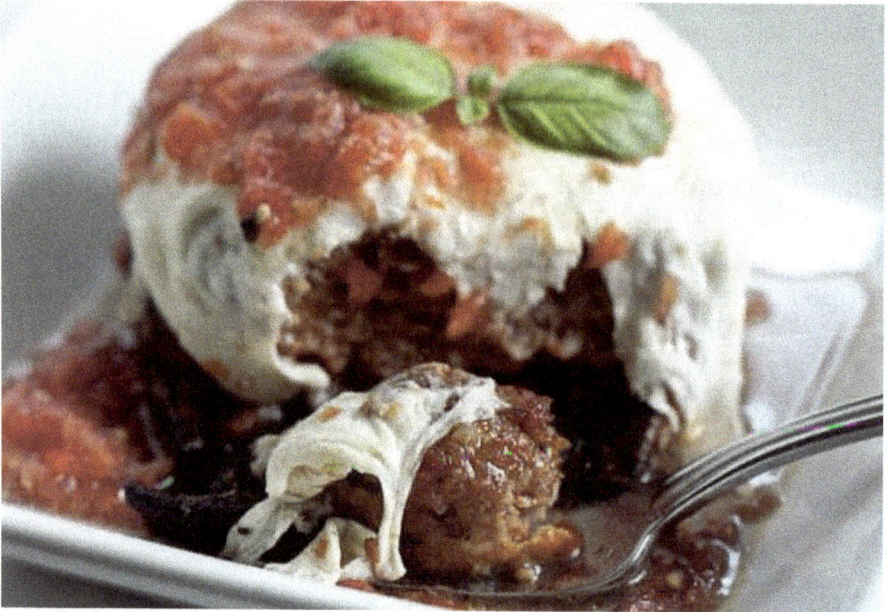

Puri Bread

Preparation time: 10 minutes

Cooking time: 5 minutes

Servings: 6

Ingredients:

· 1 cup almond flour, sifted

· ½ cup of warm water

· 2 tablespoons clarified butter

· 1 cup olive oil for frying

· Salt to taste

Directions:

1. Salt the water and add the flour.

2. Make a well in the center of the dough and pour warm clarified butter.

3. Knead the dough and let it stand for 15 minutes, covered.

4. Shape into 6 balls.

5. Flatten the balls into 6 thin rounds, using a rolling pin.

6. Heat enough oil to completely cover a round frying pan.

7. Place a puri in it when hot.

8. Fry for 20 seconds on each side.

9. Place on a paper towel.

10. Repeat with the rest of the puri and serve.

Nutrition:

•Calories: 106

•Fat: 3 g

•Carbs: 6 g Protein: 3 g

Breakfast Bread for keto diet

Preparation time: 15 minutes

Cooking time: 40 minutes

Servings: 16 slices

Ingredients:

· ½ teaspoon xanthan gum

· ½ teaspoon salt

· 2 tablespoons coconut oil

· ½ cup butter, melted

· 1 teaspoon baking powder

· 2 cups of almond flour

· 7 eggs

Directions:

1. Preheat the oven to 355°F.

2. Beat eggs in a bowl on high for 2 minutes.

3. Add coconut oil and butter to the eggs and continue to beat.

4. Line a loaf pan with baking paper and pour the beaten eggs.

5. Pour in the rest of the ingredients and mix until it becomes thick.

6. Bake until a toothpick comes out clean, about 40 to 45 minutes.

Nutrition:

· Calories: 234

· Fat: 23 g

· Carbohydrates: 1 g

· Protein: 7 g

French Bread

Preparation time: 2 hours 30 minutes

Cooking time: 30 minutes

Servings: 14

Ingredients:

· 1 1/3 cups warm water

· 1 ½ tablespoons olive oil

· 1 ½ teaspoons salt

· 2 tablespoons sugar

· 4 cups all-purpose flour; or bread flour

· 2 teaspoons yeast

Directions:

1. Put the warm water in your bread machine first.

2. Next put in the olive oil, then the salt, and finally the sugar. Make sure to follow that exact order. Then put in the flour, make sure to cover the liquid ingredients.

3. In the center of the flour make a small well, make sure the well doesn't go down far enough to touch the liquid. Put the yeast in the well.

4. Set the bread machine to the French Bread Cycle.

5. After 5 minutes of kneading, check on the dough. If the dough is stiff and dry add ½ - 1 tablespoon of water until the dough becomes a soft ball.

6. If the dough is too wet, add 1 tablespoon of flour until the right consistency is reached. Let the bread cool for 10 minutes before slicing.

Nutrition:

· Calories: 121

· Fiber: 1.1 g

· Fat: 1.9 g

· Carbohydrates: 2.9 g

· Protein: 3.9 g

Mug Bread for keto diet

Preparation time: 6 minutes

Cooking time: 4 minutes

Servings: 2

Ingredients:

· 1 pinch garlic powder

· 1 pinch pink salt

· 1 pinch onion powder

· 1 pinch black pepper

· 2 tablespoons water

· 1 pinch dried parsley

· ½ teaspoon baking powder

· 1 egg

· 2 tablespoons coconut flour

· 1 tablespoons butter, melted

· ½ cup whipping cream

· ¼ cup cheddar cheese

Directions:

1.Mix baking powder, coconut flour, garlic powder, onion powder, parsley, salt, and black pepper in a bowl.

2.Add cream, butter, water, Cheddar cheese, and egg and mix well.

3.Transfer batter into a mug and place it in a microwave oven.

4.Microwave for 4 minutes and remove.

5.Cool and serve.

Nutrition:

· Calories: 259

· Fat: 22.7 g

· Carbohydrates: 7.1 g

· Protein: 8.1 g

Carrot Polenta Loaf

Preparation time: 5 minutes

Cooking time: 3 hours

Servings: 1 loaf

Ingredients:

· 10 oz. lukewarm water

· 2 tablespoons extra-virgin olive oil

· 1 teaspoon salt

· 1 ½ tablespoons sugar

· 1 ½ tablespoons dried thyme

· 1 ½ cups freshly-grated carrots

· 1/2 cup yellow cornmeal

· 1 cup light rye flour

· 2 ½ cups bread flour

· 3 teaspoons instant active dry yeast

Direction:

1.Add all ingredients to the machine pan.

2.Select Dough setting.

3.When the cycle is completed, turn dough onto a lightly floured surface

4.Knead the dough and shape into an oval; cover with plastic wrap and let it rest for 10 to 15 minutes.

5.After resting, turn the bottom side up and flatten.

6.Fold the top 1/3 of the way to the bottom. Then fold the bottom a 1/3 of the way over the top. Press dough with the palm of your hand to make an indent in the center, and then fold the top completely down to the bottom, sealing the seam.

7.Preheat oven to 400°F.

8.Dust a baking sheet with cornmeal, place dough on and cover in a warm place to rise for 20 minutes.

9.After rising, make 3 deep diagonal slashes on the top and brush the top of the bread with cold water.

10. Bake for 20 to 25 minutes or until nicely browned

Nutrition:

· Calories: 146

· Total fat: 2 g (0 g sat. fat)

· Carbohydrates: 27 g

· Fiber: 2 g

· Protein: 3.9 g

Parmesan Italian Bread

Preparation time: 16 minutes

Cooking time: 15 minutes

Servings : 10

Ingredients:

· 1 1/3 cup warm water

· 2 tablespoons olive oil

· 2 cloves of garlic, crushed

· 1 tablespoon basil

· 1 tablespoon oregano

· 1 tablespoon parsley

· 2 cups almond flour

· 1 tablespoon inulin

· ½ cup Parmesan cheese, grated

· 1 teaspoon active dry yeast

Directions:

1.Pour all wet ingredients into the bread machine pan.

2.Add all dry ingredients to the pan.

3.Set the bread machine to French bread.

4.When the bread is done, remove the bread machine pan from the bread machine.

5.Let it cool slightly before transferring to a cooling rack.

6.You can store your bread for up to 7 days.

Nutrition:

· Calories: 150

· Carbohydrates: 14 g

· Protein: 5 g

· Fat: 5 g

Almond Sweet Bread for keto diet

Preparation time: 10 minutes

Cooking time: 50 minutes

Servings: 14

Ingredients:

· 2 ¼ cups almond flour

· 2 eggs

· 2 tablespoons ground flaxseed

· ¼ teaspoon ground star anise

· ¼ teaspoon ginger powder

· 1 teaspoon baking powder

· ½ teaspoon xanthan gum

· ½ cup heavy cream

· ½ cup sugar substitute

· ½ cup butter

Directions:

1.Melt the butter in a pan. Add heavy cream and sugar substitute. Stir until mixed well. Remove from the heat and let it cool.

2.Place the rest of the dry ingredients in a bowl and whisk. Pour in the cooled cream and butter mix. Add 2 eggs and mix.

3.Line bread in with parchment paper and pour the bread dough.

4.Bake at 350°F for 45 to 50 minutes.

5.Remove, cool, and serve.

Nutrition:

· Calories: 206

· Fat: 19.8 g

· Carbohydrates: 2.3 g

· Protein: 5.2 g

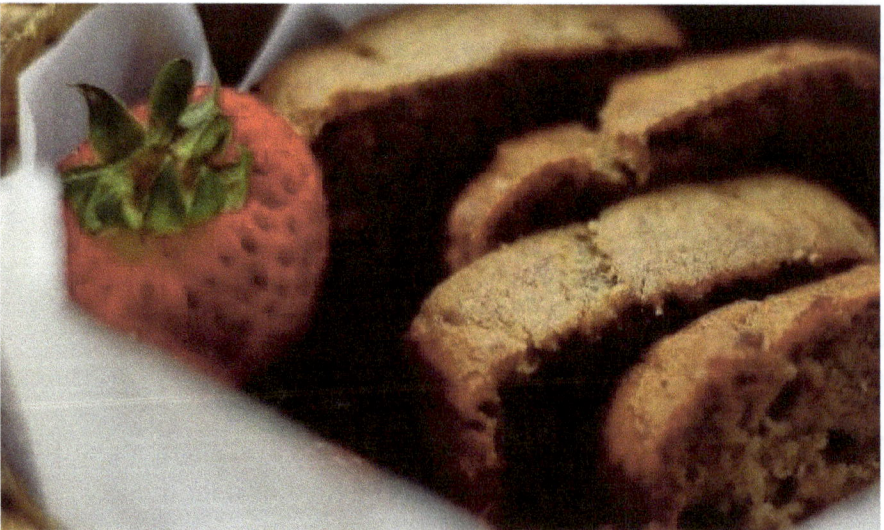

Zucchini bread with walnuts

Preparation time: 4 minutes

Cooking time: 15 minutes

Servings : 12

Ingredients:

· 2 ½ cups almond flour

· ½ cup olive oil

· 1.5 cups erythritol

· 1 teaspoon vanilla extract

· ½ teaspoon nutmeg

· 3 large eggs

· 1 ½ teaspoons baking powder

· 1 cup grated zucchinis

· 1 teaspoon cinnamon

· ¼ teaspoon ginger

· ½ teaspoon salt

· ½ cup walnuts, chopped

Directions:

1.Grate zucchini and use cheesecloth to squeeze excess water out and set aside.

2.Mix eggs, vanilla extract, and oil in the bread machine pan.

3.Add almond flour, ginger, erythritol, salt, nutmeg, baking powder, and cinnamon.

4.Add the zucchini to the bread machine pan and top with walnuts.

5.Set bread machine to Gluten-free.

6.When the bread is done, remove the bread machine pan from the bread machine.

7.Let it cool slightly before transferring to a cooling rack.

8.The bread can be stored for up to 5 days on the counter and for up to 3 months in the freezer.

Nutrition:

· Calories: 160

· Carbohydrates: 3 g

· Fats: 16 g

· Protein: 4 g

Greek Olive Bread

Preparation time: 15 minutes

Cooking time: 15 minutes

Servings : 20

Ingredients:

· 4 eggs

· 5 tablespoons ground flaxseed

· 2 teaspoons psyllium powder

· 2 tablespoons apple cider vinegar

· 1 teaspoon baking soda

· 1 teaspoon salt

· ½ cup sour cream

· ½ cup olive oil

· 1.8 oz. black olives, chopped

· 1 teaspoon ground rosemary

· 1 ½ cups almond flour

· 1 teaspoon dried basil

Directions:

1.Beat eggs in a mixing bowl for about 5 minutes. Add olive oil slowly while you continue to beat the eggs. Add in sour cream and apple cider vinegar and continue to beat for another 5 minutes.

2.Mix all the remaining ingredients together in a separate smaller bowl.

3.Place all wet ingredients into the bread machine pan.

4.Add the remaining ingredients to the bread pan.

5.Set bread machine to the French setting.

6.When the bread is done, remove the bread machine pan from the bread machine.

7.Let it cool slightly before transferring to a cooling rack.

8.The bread can be stored for up to 7 days on the counter.

Nutrition:

· Calories: 150

· Carbohydrates: 3 g

· Protein: 3 g

· Fat: 14 g

Veggie Loaf

Preparation time: 20 minutes

Cooking time: 15 minutes

Servings : 20

Ingredients:

· 1/3 cup coconut flour

· 2 tablespoons chia seeds

· 2 tablespoons psyllium husk powder

· ¼ cup sunflower seeds

· ¼ cup pumpkin seeds

· 2 tablespoons flax seed

· 1 cup almond flour

· 1 cup zucchini, grated

· 4 eggs

· ¼ cup coconut oil, melted

· 1 tablespoon paprika

· 2 teaspoons cumin

· 2 teaspoons baking powder

· 2 teaspoons salt

Directions:

1.Grate carrots and zucchini; use cheesecloth to squeeze excess water out, set it aside.

2.Mix eggs and coconut oil into bread machine pan.

3.Add the remaining ingredients to the bread pan.

4.Set bread machine to Quick bread setting.

5.When the bread is done, remove the bread machine pan from the bread machine.

6.Let it cool slightly before transferring to a cooling rack.

7.You can store your veggie loaf bread for up to 5 days in the refrigerator, or it can also be sliced and stored in the freezer for up to 3 months.

Nutrition:

· Calories: 150

· Carbohydrates: 3 g

· Protein: 3 g

· Fat: 14 g

Pumpkin Bread Loaf for keto diet

Preparation time: 7 minutes

Cooking time: 25 min

Servings: 14

Ingredients:

· 3 large eggs

· ½ cup olive oil

· 1 teaspoon vanilla concentrate

· 2 1/2 cups almond flour

· 1 1/2 cups erythritol

· ½ teaspoon salt

· 1 1/2 teaspoons preparing powder

· ½ teaspoon nutmeg

· 1 teaspoon ground cinnamon

· ¼ teaspoon ground ginger

· 1 cup ground zucchini

· ½ cup hacked pecans

Directions:

1.Preheat stove to 350°F. Whisk together the eggs, oil, and vanilla concentrate. Set it aside.

2.In another bowl, combine the almond flour, erythritol, salt, heating powder, nutmeg, cinnamon, and ginger. Set it aside.

3.Using a cheesecloth or paper towel, dry the zucchini and crush out.

4.Then, whisk the zucchini into the bowl with the eggs.

5.Slowly add the dry ingredients into the egg blend and with a hand blender, mix until completely combined.

6.Lightly shower a 9x5 portion dish, and spoon in the zucchini bread blend.

7.Then, spoon in the hacked pecans over the zucchini bread. Press pecans into the hitter using a spatula.

8.Bake for 60-70 minutes at 350°F or until the pecans on top look sautéed.

Nutrition:

· Cal: 70

· Carbohydratess: 6 g

· Net Carbohydrates: 2.5 g

· Fiber: 6.5 g

· Fat: 7 g

Garlic, Herb, and Cheese Bread

Preparation time: 5 minutes

Cooking time: 45 minutes

Servings : 12

Ingredients:

· ½ cup ghee

· 6 eggs

· 2 cups almond flour

· 1 teaspoon baking powder

· ½ teaspoon xanthan gum

· 1 cup Cheddar cheese, shredded

· 1 tablespoon garlic powder

· 1 tablespoon parsley

· ½ tablespoon oregano

· ½ teaspoon salt

Directions:

1.Lightly beat eggs and ghee before pouring into the bread machine pan.

1.Add the remaining ingredients to the pan.

2.Set bread machine to Gluten-free.

3.When the bread is done, remove the bread machine pan from the bread machine.

4.Let it cool slightly before transferring to a cooling rack.

5.You can store your bread for up to 5 days in the refrigerator.

Nutrition:

· Calories: 156

· Carbohydrates: 4 g

· Fats: 13 g

· Sugar: 4 g

· Protein: 5 g

Simple bread for keto diet

Preparation time: 3 minutes

Cooking time: 15 minutes

Servings: 8

Ingredients:

· 3 cups almond flour

· 2 tablespoons inulin

· 1 tablespoon whole milk

· ½ teaspoon salt

· 2 teaspoons active yeast

· 1 ¼ cups warm water

· 1 tablespoon olive oil

Directions:

1.Use a small mixing bowl to combine all dry ingredients, except for the yeast.

2.In the bread machine pan, add all wet ingredients.

3.Add all dry ingredients, from the small mixing bowl, into the bread machine pan. Top with the yeast.

4.Set the bread machine to the Basic bread setting.

5.When the bread is done, remove the bread machine pan from the bread machine.

6.Let it cool slightly before transferring to a cooling rack.

7.The bread can be stored for up to 5 days on the counter and for up to 3 months in the freezer.

Nutrition:

· Carbohydrates: 4 g

· Fats: 7 g

· Protein: 3 g

· Calories: 85

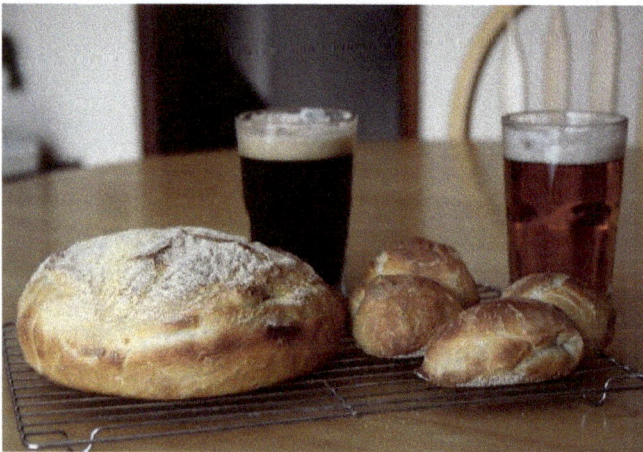

Sourdough Bread

Preparation time: 6 minutes

Cooking time: 15 minutes

Servings : 10

Ingredients:

· ½ cup almond flour

· ½ cup coconut flour

· ½ cup ground flaxseed

· 1/3 cup psyllium husk powder

· 1 teaspoon baking soda

· 1 teaspoon Himalayan salt

· 2 eggs

· 6 egg whites

· ¾ cup buttermilk

· ¼ cup apple cider vinegar

· ½ cup warm water

Directions:

1.Combine the flours, flaxseed, psyllium husk, baking soda, and salt into a bowl, mix together, and set aside.

2.Place eggs, egg whites, and buttermilk into bread machine baking pan.

3.Add dry ingredients on top, and then pour over the vinegar and warm water.

4.Set bread machine to French setting (or a similar longer setting).

5.Check dough during the kneading process to see if more water may be needed.

6.When the bread is done, remove the bread machine pan from the bread machine.

7.Let it cool slightly before transferring to a cooling rack.

8.The bread can be stored for up to 10 days in the fridge or for 3 months in the freezer.

Nutrition:

· Calories: 85

· Carbohydrates: 4 g

· Fats: 4 g

· Protein: 6 g

Garlic Bread

Preparation time: 2 hours

Cooking time: 15 minutes

Servings: 6

Ingredients:

· 5 oz. beef

· 15 oz. almond flour

· 5 oz. rye flour

· 1 onion

· 3 teaspoons dry yeast

· 5 tablespoons olive oil

· 1 tablespoon sugar

· Sea salt

· Ground black pepper

Directions:

1.Pour the warm water into the 15 oz. of the almond flour and rye flour and leave overnight.

2.Chop the onions and cut the beef into cubes.

3.Fry the onions until clear and golden brown, then mix in the bacon and fry on low heat for 20 minutes until soft.

4.Combine the yeast with the warm water, mixing until smooth consistency, and then combine the yeast with the flour, salt and sugar—but don't forget to mix and knead well.

5.Add in the fried onions with the beef and black pepper, and mix well.

6.Pour some oil into a bread machine and place the dough into the bread maker. Cover the dough with the towel and leave for 1 hour.

7.Close the lid and turn the bread machine on the Basic/white bread program.

8.Bake the bread until the medium crust and after the bread is ready, take it out and leave for 1 hour covered with the towel. Only then you can slice the bread.

Nutrition:

· Carbohydrates: 6 g

· Fats: 21 g

· Protein: 13 g

· Calories: 299

Cajun Veggie Loaf

Preparation time: 15 minutes

Cooking time: 15 minutes

Servings : 12

Ingredients:

· ½ cup water

· ¼ cup onion, chopped

· ½ cup green bell pepper, chopped

· 2 teaspoons garlic, chopped finely

· 2 teaspoons ghee

· 2 cups almond flour

· 1 tablespoon inulin

· 1 teaspoon Cajun seasoning

· 1 teaspoon active dry yeast

Directions:

1.Add water and ghee to the bread machine pan.

2.Add in the remaining ingredients.

3.Set bread machine to the Basic setting.

4.When done, remove from the bread machine and allow cooling before slicing.

5.Let it cool slightly before transferring to a cooling rack.

6.You can store your bread for up to 5 days in the refrigerator.

Nutrition:

· Calories: 101

· Carbohydrates: 6g

· Protein: 4 g

· Fat: 8 g

Pumpkin Bread

Preparation time: 5 minutes

Cooking time: 15 minutes

Servings : 8

Ingredients:

· 6 eggs

· 8 tablespoons butter, melted

· 2 cups almond flour

· 2 teaspoons baking powder

· ¼ teaspoon ground allspice

· ¼ teaspoon ground cloves

· ¼ teaspoon ground nutmeg

· ½ cup erythritol

· ½ cup pumpkin puree

· 1 teaspoon cinnamon

· 3 tablespoons sour cream

· 1 teaspoon vanilla

· 2 tablespoons heavy cream

Directions:

1.In the bread machine pan, add all the wet ingredients.

2.Then add the dry ingredients on top.

3.Set the bread machine to the Gluten-free bread setting.

4.When the bread is done, remove the bread machine pan from the bread machine.

5.Let it cool slightly before transferring to a cooling rack.

6.The bread can be stored for up to 5 days on the counter.

Nutrition:

· Calories: 220

· Carbohydrates: 14 g

· Fats: 21 g

· Protein: 6 g

Pumpkin and Sunflower Seed Bread

Preparation time: 8 minutes

Cooking time: 15 minutes

Servings : 10

Ingredients:

· ½ cup ground psyllium husk

· ½ cup chia seeds

· ½ cup pumpkin seeds

· ½ cup sunflower seeds

· 2 tablespoons ground flaxseed

· 1 teaspoon baking soda

· ¼ teaspoon salt

· 3 tablespoons coconut oil, melted

· 1 ¼ cups egg whites

· ½ cup almond milk

Directions:

1.Place all wet ingredients into the bread machine pan first.

2.Add dry ingredients.

3.Set bread machine to the Gluten-free setting.

4.When the bread is done, remove the bread machine pan from the bread machine.

5.Let it cool slightly before transferring to a cooling rack.

6.You can store your bread for up to 5 days in the refrigerator.

Nutrition:

· Calories: 155

· Carbohydrates: 4 g

· Fats: 8 g

· Sugar: 3 g

· Protein: 5 g

Rosemary & Garlic Coconut Flour Bread

Preparation time: 20 minutes

Cooking time: 45 min

Ingredients:

· ½ cup Coconut flour

· 1 sticks margarine (8 tablespoon)

· 6 large eggs

· 1 teaspoon heating powder

· 2 teaspoons Dried Rosemary

· ½ -1 teaspoon garlic powder

· ½ teaspoon Onion powder

· ¼ teaspoon Pink Himalayan Salt

Directions:

1.Add dry ingredients (coconut flour, heating powder, onion, garlic, rosemary, and salt) to a bowl and put them in a safe spot.

2.Add 6 eggs to a different bowl and beat with a hand blender until you get see rises at the top.

3.Melt the stick of margarine in the microwave and gradually add it to the eggs as you beat with the hand blender.

4.When wet and dry ingredients are completely consolidated in isolated dishes, gradually add the dry ingredients to the wet ingredients as you blend in with the hand blender.

5.Oil an 8x4 portion dish and empty the blend into it equitably.

6.Heat at 350 °F for 40-50 minutes (time will change contingent upon your broiler).

7.Let it rest for 10 minutes before removing it from the container. Cut up and enjoy it with spread or toasted!

Nutrition:

· Calories: 21

· Fat: 4.7 g

· Carbohydrates: 44.2 g

· Protein: 0

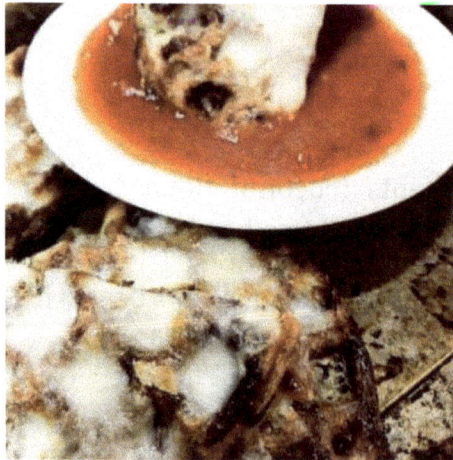

Best Garlic Bread for keto diet

Preparation time: 10

Cooking time: 15

Ingredients:

Garlic and Herb Compound Butter:

· ½ cup mellowed unsalted margarine (113 g/4 oz.)

· ½ teaspoon salt (I like pink Himalayan salt)

· 1/4 teaspoon ground dark pepper

· 2 tablespoons additional virgin olive oil (30 ml)

· 4 garlic cloves, squashed

· 2 tablespoons naturally slashed parsley or 2 teaspoon dried parsley

Topping:

· ½ cup ground Parmesan cheddar (45 g/1.6 oz.)

· 2 tablespoons crisp parsley

Discretionary: sprinkle with additional virgin olive oil

Alternative options:

· Extreme Keto Buns

· Nut-Free Keto Buns

· Psyllium-Free Keto Buns

· Flax-Free Keto Bread

Directions:

1.Set up the Keto sourdough rolls by following this formula (you can make 8 standard or 16 smaller than usual loaves).

2.Set up the garlic margarine (or some other seasoned spread). Ensure every one of the ingredients has been set aside at room temperature before blending them in a medium bowl.

3.Cut the prepared rolls down the middle and spread the enhanced margarine over every half (1–2 teaspoons for each piece).

4.Sprinkle with ground Parmesan and put back in the stove to fresh up for a couple of more minutes.

5.At the point when done, remove from the stove. Alternatively, sprinkle with some olive oil and serve while still warm.

Nutrition:

· Calories: 270

· Fat: 15 g

· Fiber: 3 g

· Carbohydrates: 5 g

· Protein: 9 g

Cheesy Sesame Bread

Preparation time: 5 minutes

Cooking time: 30 minutes

Servings: 8

Ingredients:

· 1 teaspoon sesame seeds

· 1 teaspoon baking powder

· 1 teaspoon salt

· 2 tablespoons ground psyllium husk powder

· 1 cup almond flour

· 4 tablespoons sesame or olive oil

· 7 ounces cream cheese

· 4 eggs

· Sea salt

Directions:

1.Preheat the oven to 400°F.

2.Beat the eggs until fluffy. Add cream cheese and oil until combined well.

3.Set the sesame seeds aside and add the remaining ingredients.

4.Grease a baking tray. Spread the dough in the greased baking tray. Allow it to stand for 5 minutes.

5.Baste dough with oil and top with a sprinkle of sesame seeds and a little sea salt.

6.Bake in the oven at 400°F until the top is golden brown— about 30 minutes.

Nutrition:

· Calories: 282

· Fat: 26 g

· Carbohydrates: 2 g

· Protein: 7 g

Cheese Blend Bread

Preparation time: 45 minutes

Cooking time: 20 minutes

Servings: 12

Ingredients:

· 5 oz. cream cheese

· 1/4 cup g hee

· 2/3 cup almond flour

· 1/4 cup coconut flour

· 3 tablespoons whey protein, unflavored

· 2 teaspoons baking powder

· 1/2 teaspoon Himalayan salt

· 1/2 cup Parmesan cheese, shredded

· 3 tablespoons water

· 3 eggs

· 1/2 cup m ozzarella cheese , shredded

Directions:

1.Place wet ingredients into bread machine pan.

93

2.Add dry ingredients.

3.Set the bread machine to the Gluten-free setting.

4.When the bread is done, remove the bread machine pan from the bread machine.

5.Let it cool slightly before transferring to a cooling rack.

6.You can store your bread for up to 5 days.

Nutrition:

· Calories: 132

· Carbohydrates: 4 g

· Protein: 6 g

· Fat: 8 g

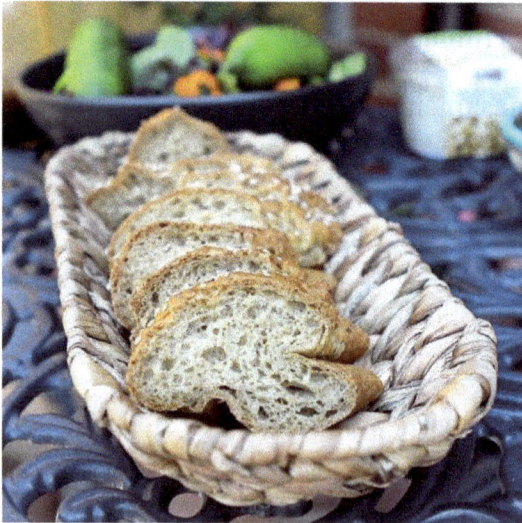

Lemon & Rosemary Low Carb Shortbread

Preparation time: 5 minutes

Cooking time: 20 min

Servings: 6

Ingredients:

· 6 tablespoons margarine

· 2 cups almond flour

· 1/3 cup granulated Splenda (or other granulated sugar)

· 1 tablespoon naturally ground lemon get-up-and-go

· 4 teaspoons crisp pressed lemon juice

· 1 teaspoon vanilla concentrate

· 2 teaspoons rosemary

· ½ teaspoon preparing pop

· ½ teaspoon preparing powder

Directions:

1.In a large blending bowl, measure out 2 cups of almond flour, ½ teaspoon heating powder, and ½ teaspoon preparing pop. Add 1/3 cup Splenda, or other granulated sugar in the blend. Put in a safe spot.

2.Zest your lemon with a Microplane until you have 1 Tablespoon lemon get-up-and-go. Squeeze a large portion of the lemon to get 4 teaspoon lemon juice.

3.In the microwave, melt 6 Tablespoon of margarine and afterward include 1 teaspoon vanilla concentrate.

4.Transfer your almond flour and sugar to a little blending bowl. Put your spread, lemon get-up-and-go, lemon squeeze, and slashed rosemary into the now-empty large blending bowl. Add the almond flour once more into the wet blend gradually, mixing as you go. Continue blending until all the almond flour is added back.

5.Wrap the mixture firmly in cling wrap.

6.Place the enveloped batter in the cooler for 30 minutes, or until hard.

7.Preheat your stove to 350°F, take out the batter, and unwrap it.

8.Cut your batter in ~1/2" increases with a sharp blade. In the event that this blade isn't sharp, it will cause the batter to disintegrate. On the off chance that the mixture is as yet disintegrating, that implies it needs additional time in the cooler.

9.Grease a treat sheet with salted margarine and place your treats onto it.

Nutrition:

· Calories: 100

· Carbohydrates: 2 g

· Net Carbohydrates: 5.5 g

Cauliflower Bread with Garlic & Herbs

Preparation time: 9 minutes

Cooking time: 26 min

Servings: 12

Ingredients:

· 3 cups cauliflower ("riced" utilizing food processor*)

· 10 large eggs (isolated)

· 1/4 teaspoon cream of tartar (discretionary)

· 1 ¼ cups coconut flour

· 1 ½ teaspoons sans gluten heating powder

· 1 teaspoon sea salt

· 6 teaspoons butter (unsalted, estimated strong, then softened; can utilize ghee for sans dairy)

· 6 cloves garlic (minced)

· 1 teaspoon fresh rosemary (slashed)

· 1 teaspoon fresh parsley (slashed)

Directions:

1.Preheat the broiler to 350 °F (177 ° C). Line a 9x5 in (23x13 cm) portion skillet with material paper.

2.Steam the riced cauliflower. You can do this in the microwave (cooked for 3–4 minutes, shrouded in plastic) or in a steamer bin over water on the stove (line with cheesecloth if the openings in the steamer container are too big, and steam for a couple of moments). The two different ways, steam until the cauliflower is soft. Let the cauliflower cool enough to deal with.

3.Meanwhile, use a hand blender to beat the egg whites and cream of tartar until solid pinnacles structure.

4.Place the coconut flour, preparing powder, ocean salt, egg yolks, melted margarine, garlic, and 1/4 of the whipped egg whites in a food processor.

5.When the cauliflower has cooled enough to deal with, envelop it with a kitchen towel and press a few times to dry much wet as could reasonably be expected. (This is significant — the final product ought to be dry and bunch together.) Add the cauliflower to the food processor. Pulse until all-around joined. (Blend will be thick and somewhat brittle.)

6.Add the rest of the egg whites to the food processor. Overlay in only a bit, to make it simpler to process. Pulse a couple of times until simply consolidated. (Blend will be cushioned.) Fold in the hacked parsley and rosemary. (Don't over-blend to avoid separating the egg whites excessively.)

7.Transfer the layer into the lined heating skillet. Smooth the top and adjust somewhat. Whenever wanted, you can squeeze more herbs into the top (discretionary).

8.Bake for around 45-50 minutes, until the top is brilliant. Cool totally before removing and cutting .

How To Make Buttered Low Carb Garlic Bread (discretionary) :

Top cuts liberally with spread, minced garlic, crisp parsley, and a little ocean salt. Prepare in a preheated stove at 450 °F (233 °C) for around 10 minutes. On the off chance that you need it progressively sautéed, place in the oven for several minutes.

Nutrition:

· Calories: 70

· Carbohydrates: 4 g

· Net Carbohydrates: 2.5 g

· Fiber: 4.5 g

· Fat: 15 g

· Protein: 4 g

Cheesy Garlic Bread

Preparation time: 30 minutes

Cooking time: 20 minutes

Servings: 10

Ingredients:

· 3/4 cup mozzarella, shredded

· 1/2 cup almond flour

· 2 tablespoons cream cheese

· 1 tablespoon garlic, crushed

· 1 tablespoon parsley

· 1 teaspoon baking powder

· Salt, to taste

· 1 egg

For the toppings:

· 2 tablespoons melted butter

· 1/2 teaspoon parsley

· 1 teaspoon garlic clove, minced

Directions:

1.Mix together your topping ingredients and set aside.

2. Pour the remaining wet ingredients into the bread machine pan.

3.Add the dry ingredients.

4.Set bread machine to the Gluten-free setting.

5.When the bread is done, remove the bread machine pan from the bread machine.

6.Let it cool slightly before transferring to a cooling rack.

7.Once on a cooling rack, drizzle with the topping mix.

8.You can store your bread for up to 7 days.

Nutrition:

· Calories: 29

· Carbohydrates: 1 g

· Protein: 2 g

· Fat: 2 g

Grain-Free Tortillas Bread

Preparation time: 5 minutes

Cooking time: 20 min

Servings : 5

Ingredients:

· 96 g almond flour

· 24 g coconut flour

· 2 teaspoons thickener

· 1 teaspoon heating powder

· 1/4 teaspoon fit salt

· 2 teaspoons apple juice vinegar

· 1 egg softly beaten

· 3 teaspoons water

Directions:

1.Add almond flour, coconut flour, thickener, preparing powder, and salt to food processor. Pulse until completely joined. Note: you can, on the other hand, whisk everything in a large bowl and use the hand or stand blender to mix them.

2.Pour in apple juice vinegar while the food processor running. When it has mixed equally, pour in the egg. Then add the water, stop the food processor once the batter forms into a ball. The batter will be clingy to contact.

3.Wrap mixture in stick film and ply it through the plastic for a moment or two. Consider it somewhat like a pressure ball. Let the mixture rest for 10 minutes (and as long as three days in the refrigerator).

4.Heat a skillet (ideally) or container over medium warmth. You can test the warmth by sprinkling a couple of water beads, if the drops vanish promptly your dish is excessively hot. The beads should 'go' through the skillet.

5.With the mixture form eight balls (26g each). Put them between two sheets of material or waxed paper with a moving pin or using a tortilla press (simpler!) until each ball is 5-crawls in distance across.

6.Transfer them to a skillet and cook over medium warmth for only 3-6 seconds (significant). Flip it over promptly (using a meager spatula or blade), and keep on cooking until just daintily brilliant on each side (however with the customary roasted imprints)—30 to 40 seconds. The key isn't to overcook them, as they will never again be flexible or puff up.

7.Keep them warm enveloped by kitchen towel until serving. To rewarm, heat quickly on the two sides (not exactly a moment).

8.These tortillas are best eaten straight. Be that as it may, don't hesitate to keep some convenient mixture in your refrigerator for as long as three days, and they likewise freeze well for as long as three months.

Nutrition:

· Calories: 70 Fat: 8 g

· Carbs: 22 g Net Carbs: 2.5 g

· Fiber: 4.5g Protein: 8 g

Basil Cheese Bread

Preparation time: 5 minutes

Cooking time: 15 minutes

Servings: 10

Ingredients:

· 2 cups almond flour

· 1 cup warm water

· ½ teaspoon salt

· 1 teaspoon basil dried

· ½ cup of mozzarella shredded cheese

· ¼ teaspoon of active dry yeast

· 3 teaspoons of melted unsalted butter

· 1 teaspoon of stevia powder

Directions:

1.In a mixing container, combine the almond flour, dried basil, salt, shredded mozzarella cheese, and stevia powder.

2.Get another container, where you will combine the warm water and the melted unsalted butter.

3.As per the instructions on the manual of your machine, pour the ingredients in the bread pan, taking care to follow how to mix in the yeast.

4.Place the bread pan in the machine, and select the Sweet bread setting, together with the crust type, if available, then press Start once you have closed the lid of the machine.

5.When the bread is ready, using oven mitts, remove the bread pan from the machine. Use a stainless spatula to extract the bread from the pan and turn the pan upside down on a metallic rack where the bread will cool off before slicing it.

Nutrition:

· Calories: 124

· Fat: 8 g

· Carbohydrates: 2 g

· Protein: 11 g

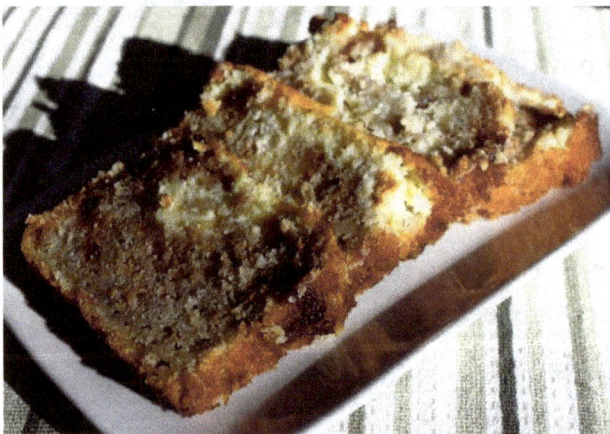

Ricotta Bread

Preparation time: 3 hours

Cooking time: 30 minutes

Servings: 10

Ingredients:

· 1/3 cup milk

· 1 cup ricotta cheese

· 2 tablespoons butter

· 1 egg

· 2 ½ tablespoons sugar

· 1 teaspoon salt

· 2 ¼ cups bread flour

· 1 ½ teaspoons yeast

Directions:

1.Put all the bread ingredients in your bread machine, in the way listed above, starting with the milk, and finishing with the yeast.

2.Make a well in the middle of the flour and place the yeast in the well. Make sure the well doesn't touch any liquid. Set the bread machine to the Basic function with the light crust.

3.Check on the dough after about 5 minutes and make sure that it's a soft ball. Add water— 1 tablespoon at a time if it's too dry— and add flour —1 tablespoon at a time if it's too wet.

4.When the bread is done, allow it cool on a wire rack.

Nutrition:

· Calories: 115

· Fiber: 1.1 g

· Fat: 6.5 g

· Carbohydrates: 3.3 g

· Protein: 8.5 g

Cauliflower Tortillas Bread

Preparation time: 6 minutes

Cooking time: 21 min

Servings: 5

Ingredients:

· 3/4 big head cauliflower (or two cups riced)

· 2 large eggs (Vegans, sub flax eggs)

· 1/4 cup cleaved crisp cilantro

· 1/2 medium lime, squeezed and zested

· Salt and pepper, to taste

Directions:

1.Preheat the stove to 375 °F., and line a heating sheet with material paper.

2.Trim the cauliflower. Cut it into little, uniform pieces, and pulses in a food processor in groups until you get a couscous-like consistency. The finely riced cauliflower should make around 2 cups pressed.

3.Place the cauliflower in a microwave-safe bowl and microwave for 2 minutes, then mix and microwave again for an additional 2 minutes. In the event that you don't use a microwave, a steamer works similarly. Place the cauliflower in a fine cheesecloth or slender dishtowel and dry up as much fluid as could be expected, being careful not to burn yourself. Dishwashing gloves are recommended as it is extremely hot.

4.In a medium bowl, whisk the eggs. Add cauliflower, cilantro, lime, salt, and pepper. Blend until all combined. With your hands, shape 6 little "tortillas" on the material paper.

5.Bake for 10 minutes, cautiously flip every tortilla, and put back to the stove for an extra 5 to 7 minutes, or until totally set. Place tortillas on a wire rack to cool marginally.

6.Heat a medium-sized skillet on medium. Place a prepared tortilla in the container, pushing down somewhat, until dark-colored —for 1 to 2 minutes on each side. Do the same way with the remaining tortillas.

Nutrition:

· Calories: 30

· Carbohydrates: 8 g

· Net Carbohydrates: 2.5 g

· Fiber: 7.5 g

· Fat: 8 g

· Protein: 10 g

Herb Focaccia Bread

Preparation time: 3.5 hours

Cooking time: 45 minutes

Servings: 8

Difficulty: Expert

Ingredients:

Dough:

· 1 cup water

· 2 tablespoons canola oil

· 1 teaspoon salt

· 1 teaspoon dried basil

· 3 cups bread flour

· 2 teaspoons bread machine yeast

Topping:

· 1 tablespoon canola oil

· ½ cup fresh basil

· 2 garlic cloves (to taste)

· 2 tablespoons grated Parmesan cheese

· 1 pinch salt

· 1 tablespoon cornmeal (optional)

Directions:

1.Put all the bread ingredients in your bread machine, in the way they are listed above —starting with the water and finishing with the yeast. Make a well in the middle of the flour and place the yeast in the well. Make sure the well doesn't touch any liquid. Set the bread machine to the Dough function.

2.Check on the dough after about 5 minutes and make sure that it's a soft ball. Add water —1 tablespoon at a time if it's too dry, and add flour— 1 tablespoon at a time if it's too wet.

3.When the dough is ready, put it on a lightly floured hard surface. Cover the dough and let it rest for 10 minutes.

4.While the dough is resting, chop the garlic and basil, grease a 13x9 inch pan, and evenly sprinkle with cornmeal on top of it.

5.Once the dough has rested, press it into the greased pan. Drizzle oil on the dough and evenly sprinkle with the salt Parmesan, garlic, and basil.

Nutrition:

· Calories: 108

· Carbohydrates: 37.4 g

· Fiber: 1.6 g

· Fat: 7.3 g

· Protein: 7.7 g